Coming Home:

A Discharge Manual For Families Of Persons With A Brain Injury

Dana S. DeBoskey, Ph.D., Editor

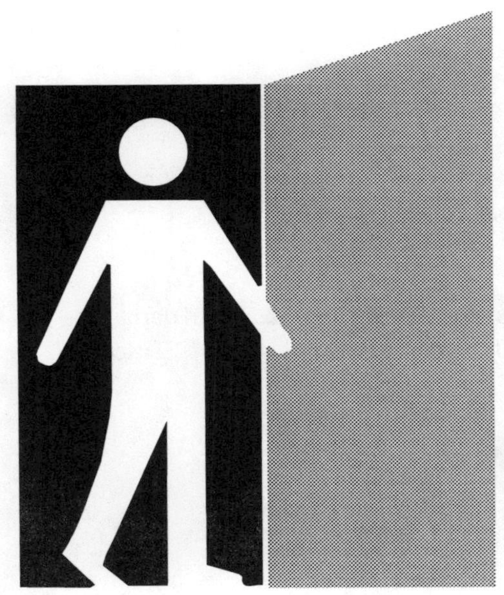

AF531262

© Copyright 1996

No part of this book may be reproduced, stored in a retrieval system, or transmitted, by any means, electronic or mechanical, including photocopying, without written permission from the publisher.

Printed in the United States of America on acid free paper. ∞

Library of Congress Cataloging-in-Publication Data
DeBoskey, Dana S.
Coming home : a discharge manual for families of persons with a brain injury / by Dana S. DeBoskey.
p. cm.
ISBN 1-882855-34-5
1. Brain damage--Patients--Rehabilitation. 2. Brain damage--Psychological aspects. 3. Adjustment (Psychology). I. Title.
RC387.5.D437 1996
617.4'8103--dc20

96-7502
CIP

This manual was developed and produced
by DeBoskey and Associates, Tampa, Florida.
Other volumes by DeBoskey and Associates published
by HDI include:

An Educational Challenge: Meeting the Needs of Students With Brain Injury

Working After Brain Injury: What Can I Do?

Pain: Making Life Liveable

For a complete catalog of
HDI's brain injury resources contact:

HDI Publishers
P.O. Box 131401
Houston, TX 77219
Toll Free (800) 321-7037
Fax (713) 956-2288

DEDICATION

To the Coxes and their son, Rob, who opened my eyes to the need for a "going home" manual. And to the multitude of families who shared with me the fears and anxieties of bringing their loved one home.

TABLE OF CONTENTS

PREFACE

Patients who are brain injured obtain constant and specifically skilled rehabilitation services when they are involved in a residential program, either acute or post acute. Pending discharge, all professionals, including case managers, therapists, social workers, and psychologists, make a concentrated effort to provide the family and/or primary caretaker with all the information needed to effectively manage this individual in the home setting. Many man hours are involved in planning a smooth discharge. If this is the case, why do many families feel so ill prepared once they are ultimately on their own? Is it the fault of the therapists for not telling them what it would really be like? Did they think the family would not take the patient home if they knew the truth? Or...is it the family's fault for not listening when the needed information was given to them? Did the family not show up when family education help was offered? Did the family deny that they needed help, thinking that the injured patient would not show those awful behaviors at home?

More often than not it involves a combination of factors and cannot be attributed to any single issue. Nevertheless, no matter what the origin, families continue to have significant adjustment problems when the patient leaves the rehabilitation facility. Some are lucky enough to have excellent outpatient services that they can consult anytime of the day. Others are out there almost on their own. No matter where the family falls along the continuum of healthcare follow-up, they can all benefit from up-to-date knowledge and ideas regarding "what to do if..."

This manual has been written as a very practical addendum to any interdisciplinary rehabilitation effort. It is intended to cover what most families were told, as well as what they may have misinterpreted, denied, or thought was completely unnecessary in their case. It is not meant to be a replacement for appropriate follow-up, but it is sufficiently comprehensive to be helpful in those cases where follow-up services are not available. In essence, it is an effort to fill in one of the gaps that can occur in brain injury rehabilitation.

Dana S. DeBoskey, Ph.D.
April, 1996

I. INTRODUCTION

As so many people have probably indicated to you, the family is considered the key to the rehabilitation efforts. This is a big responsibility, as you well know, and there is often little written to provide you with **practical** ideas to implement, discard, revamp, or modify. The purpose of this manual is to provide you with an extensive list of ideas. Obviously, not all of them will work with your loved one. Maybe in some areas no one idea will completely solve the problem. However, it is hoped that you will be provided with information and solutions that can bring some relief.

It was the family of a loved one with a brain injury who initially asked me to write this book, and it was the opportunity to work one-on-one with families that has allowed me to test out some of the ideas presented.

One of the great difficulties in writing a book that you hope will help everyone is the wide variation in circumstances that exist from facility to facility and from milder to more severe injuries. An attempt has been made to provide something for everybody in hopes that the information can be useful to the largest number of families. If not all the suggestions are applicable to your case, read them anyway - you may be able to provide help to other families where this information does apply.

This book can be used in a variety of ways. If you are getting ready for discharge, read everything through carefully, trying to digest the main issues. If your loved one is in crisis at home, go directly to the behavior and/or behaviors that are a problem. If you are becoming overwhelmed, go to the family behavior section and obtain ideas for combating **your** problems.

There is nothing that can take the place of a supportive professional to assist you with reintegrating your loved one back into the community. If these services are available to you, do not refuse them thinking that this manual can do it all. It is only one aid to the tremendously complex job of bringing your loved one home.

Although the author is well aware that not all individuals who are brain injured are male, for the sake of simplicity the pronouns he and him are used to represent the entire population. It is hoped that this will not be offensive to anyone.

II. THE NEW PARENT SYNDROME

If you are a parent, I would like you to remember back to the early days when you brought that new baby home. Everyone was so excited about him coming home, but within a week you were worn to a frazzle trying to adjust to the new family member. Bringing your injured loved one home may actually transport you back in time in reference to the overwhelming time commitment involved in caring for a new baby.

You may be saying, “Oh it won’t be like that for us. Fred is working and can pretty much take care of himself.” Or, you may say “Fred has been in and out of two other rehab programs. We know what it is like.” The reality is that sometimes people forget and actually subconsciously block out the extreme tiredness that prevailed after discharge.

You may in fact remember quite well. In any event, get yourself mentally prepared to become a new parent. Get your life organized as much as possible so that you can minimize the added stressors. If possible, talk with other families who have recently experienced the discharge. See about a support group in your community.

EXAMPLES

1. You find that every minute of every day belongs to someone else - your time is not your own.
2. You did not realize what it would be like to assist him in the bathroom day and night.
3. You find yourself unable to rest because your mind is so full of worries about what you should be doing next.
4. You now think of a million questions that you should have asked before he left to come home.

RESOLUTIONS

1. Make sure that you have some back-up help lined up before the loved one is discharged.

2. Do not allow yourself to believe that you can take care of everything.

3. Beware if you are thinking, "There's no one I can trust to care for him while I am gone."

4. Do not allow yourself to think that your loved one should have a break and not go to outpatient therapies immediately upon coming home. If therapy has been recommended, start it as soon as possible.

5. If you find your blood pressure rising or any other symptom of increased stress, consider seeking counseling support in the community.

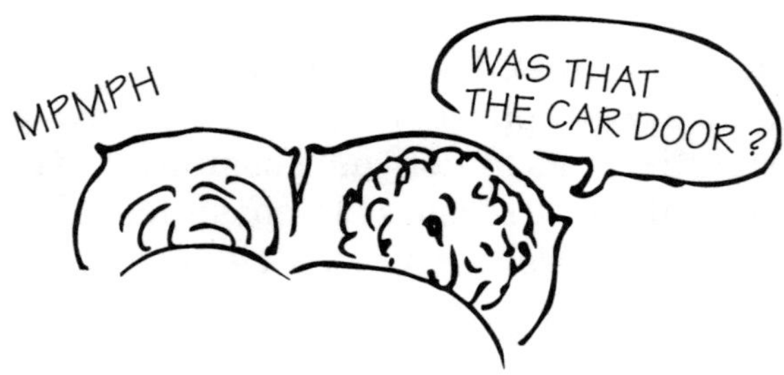

III. THE HOSPITAL SYNDROME

Your loved one may have been in an acute care rehab facility or he may be coming home from a transitional living facility whose purpose was to foster independence. In any event, there will be particular aspects of having been in a facility that will lead the individual to have certain expectations about what should happen at home.

Because patients who are brain injured sometimes distort reality or have petty remembrances about what has happened recently in the past, it is important for you to find out exactly what your loved one is capable of doing. If you start assisting or actually taking over things that he can do, you may find yourself having a difficult time of talking the individual into maintaining the independence of which he is capable.

EXAMPLES

1. The loved one expects dinner right at 5:00 p.m. regardless of what is happening at home.
2. He calls you constantly to bring him things that he is perfectly capable of getting himself.
3. The individual makes the following statements: "The nurse always reminded me of my medicine." "The life skills people always helped me get my shoes on." "The physical therapist said I need to take it easy with my exercising and not overdo it."

RESOLUTIONS

1. Do not allow the individual who is brain injured to take control - you must be the controller.

2. Get a list from all therapists about what he should be able to do at home.

3. If possible, spend a whole day going through the facility's routine so that you can see first hand about his capabilities.

4. Talk to the night crew and find out about his night habits, i.e., frequency of need to urinate, possible sleepwalking, how many times he wakes up at night.

5. In essence, find out everything possible about his routine.

6. Write down the names and numbers of the therapists so that you can call if questions come up.

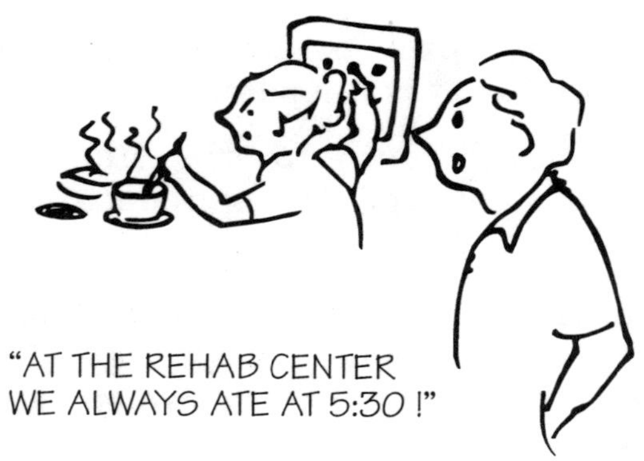

IV. NO PREFERENTIAL TREATMENT — REGARDLESS OF POSITION OR EXPERIENCE

This may not apply to you unless you work in the medical field or in the area of mental health or medical administration. For those of you in these fields, you may find that physicians, nurses, and therapists assume that you are knowledgeable in many areas of brain injury care since you work in a related field. It is analogous to someone thinking that a child psychologist's children should be under perfect control or that a counselor should be adept at managing his own stress.

You might even want to say to everybody "Forget that I am Director of Nursing at St. Joseph's Hospital - do not assume that I know the basics." Gather as much information as you can from all the therapists. They are your best source of information about what your loved one can do, cannot do, needs, or does not need. Ask lots of questions and write down what you think you might forget.

YOU ARE IN SOCIAL WORK SO YOU WON'T NEED TO SPEAK WITH OUR WORKER

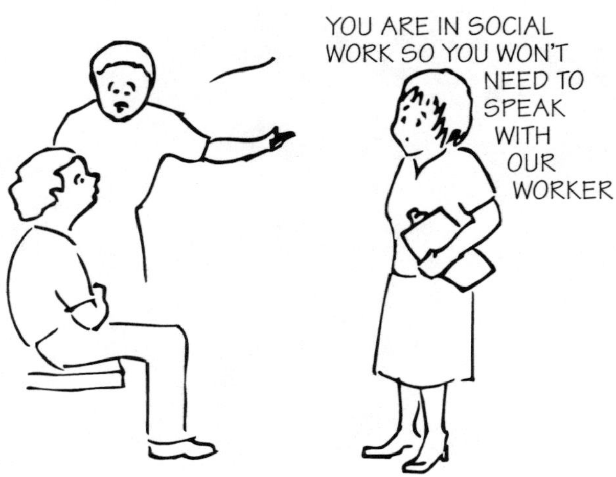

V. THE OVERPROTECTION SYNDROME — WHERE TO GO AND WHAT TO DO

Any time someone comes home from a hospital or residential facility there is a tendency to provide too much assistance, keeping with the "caretaker role." This is very counterproductive in brain injury rehabilitation. You must keep in mind that the goal is to have your loved one doing as much as he can for himself and back out into the real world. You need to facilitate all efforts at community reintegration. Start by asking the individual what he wants to do and try as much as possible to accommodate. If he rejects outings, begin a management system that will encourage him to go out into the world. You may have to begin with very short, brief excursions, such as a ride to the 7-11 to get a coke. Gradually increase these occurrences using all the help you can muster from old acquaintances and friends.

EXAMPLES

1. You avoid taking him to the mall because you are not sure how he will react.
2. You continue to cut up his meat because you do not like to see him get frustrated.
3. You will not leave him alone for more than five minutes even though the therapist told you that he could be at home on his own for one or two hours.
4. You are embarrassed by how messy he is when he eats, so you do not go out to eat at all.

RESOLUTIONS

1. Try as much as possible to include the individual in your outings.
2. Do not seriously alter your lifestyle because you think that you have to stay home and take care of your loved one.

3. Allow extra time to get ready to go anywhere with the individual. This way you will not continually feel harassed and running late.

4. Do not give in to what is easier by having therapists come to you if the person with a brain injury is capable of going to them.

5. Assume that your loved one can do a task until proven otherwise.

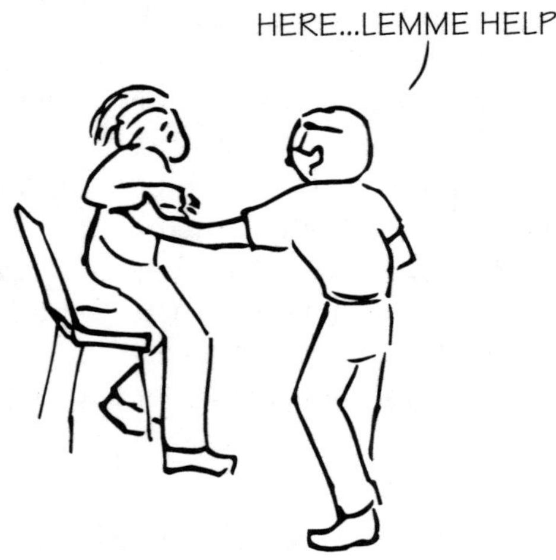

VI. THE DAILY SCHEDULE — REACTION TO CHANGE

In the rehabilitation facility there was a fairly consistent schedule. It was also quite busy and somewhat inflexible in terms of what the patient/client could choose to do or not do. Individuals who are brain injured benefit from this structure, so it will make your lives easier and the transition smoother if you have a definite schedule determined **before** the loved one is discharged.

People with brain injuries have difficulty with change, but there is no way to completely avoid this upon discharge. But, as mentioned earlier, do not allow the person three or four weeks of relaxation (inactivity) because you think, or he says, he needs a rest. You will be asking for trouble if you have to get him geared up again for a regimented schedule after weeks of "vacation." Find out exactly what he did each day and try to be as organized in his home schedule.

YAWN... GOSH ! I'M NOT
USED TO BEING UP THIS LATE !
9:00

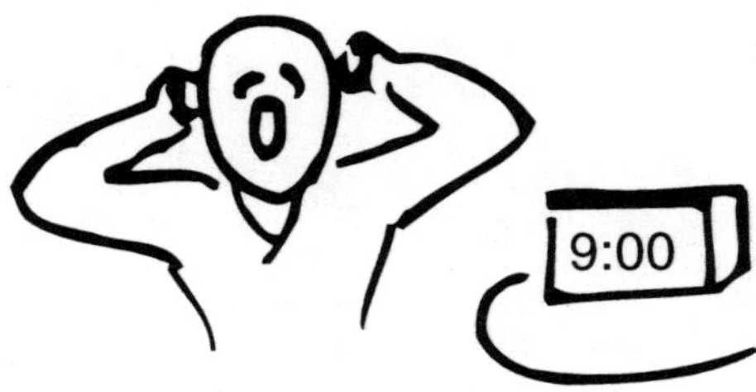

VII. ANNIVERSARY REACTION SYNDROME

If it has been less than a year since your loved one's injury, we would like to tell you about the possible anniversary reaction syndrome. As you well know, people react differently to the same situation, but there are some similarities to the thoughts that the families have as the year or two year mark approaches.

The first year anniversary is often filled with the remembrances of where you were when you were informed of the injury and all the emotional reactions and thoughts that filled your life at that time. You may have thought that you had worked through all those fears and anxieties, but they can sometimes return on the anniversary date. Another thing that can occur is that you may have had hopes that your loved one would have progressed much further by a year's time. Realizing that an entire year has passed without reaching a number of your goals may become an impetus for a depressive reaction.

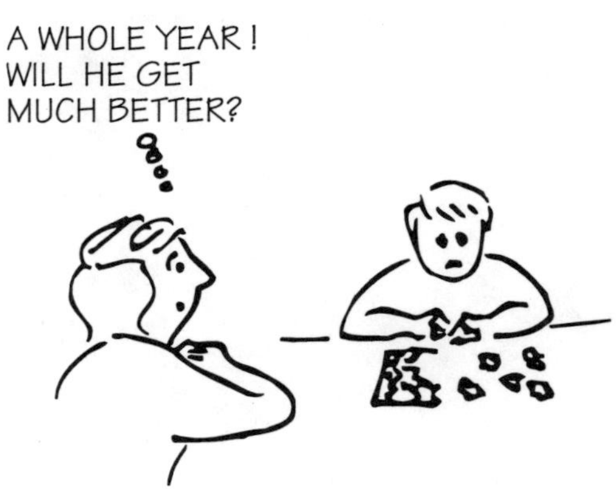

Many people make reference to the magic "Two Year Mark" when a person will have experienced most of the recovery that is to occur. It is true that a large part of the recovery takes place in the first two years, but recent research on long-term brain injury care has shown that changes can and do take place after the two year mark. These changes do not necessarily show up in better test scores, but they can certainly involve changes in psychosocial and behavioral skills. Thus, do not look on the two year time as an end to the recovery period.

VIII. PATIENT BEHAVIORS

As you have lived through your loved one's injury and recovery, you are becoming familiar with "brain injury behaviors." If it has been two years or more, you are probably very familiar, particularly if the individual has been at home for a period of time and then went to another facility due to the need for greater behavioral control or further rehabilitation. Thus, the behaviors described in this section may not be new to you. However, an attempt has been made to address these areas in light of this being a first, second, or third discharge for your family member.

If you fall into the fortunate few, you may have to concern yourself with but a few of the thirteen areas addressed. However, for the majority of you, many of these issues will still need your attention. This manual attempts to offer a menu of ideas that can be attempted in order to provide effective, efficient, and humane management of the individual who is brain injured.

You must keep in mind that the origination of most of these behaviors is due to damage to the brain. In most cases there is not a conscious effort on the individual's part to be obstinate, difficult or mean. On the other hand, if the injury has been long-standing, it is possible that inappropriate behavior has been inadvertently encouraged and that the person now acts out due to the reactions he is able to obtain from others. In any event, it is best to approach these behaviors as much as possible from a non-judgmental standpoint. It is almost always fruitless to attempt to make the person feel guilty about how he acts in hope that he will change. You may cause the guilt feelings, but a long-standing behavioral change is unlikely.

If you try to implement some of these suggestions and run up against a brick wall, it may be helpful to either get back with the behavioral specialist from the discharge facility or to hook up with a counselor (who knows brain injury!) in your community. This book is meant to be a guide to behavioral assistance - not a replacement for professional help where behaviors are out of control.

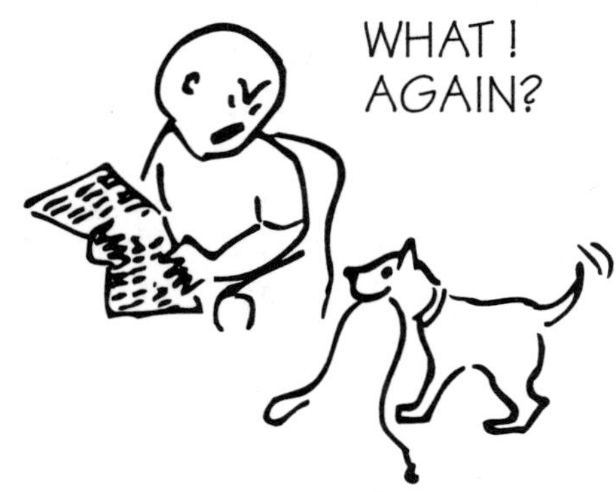

A. AGITATION / IRRITABILITY

One of the most prominent and universal personality changes after brain injury is an increase in irritability. Even those who have only been dazed by a bump on the head will often display a change in mood. For example, the once easygoing husband and father becomes someone with a short fuse. This can be very disconcerting to families who are not used to living with this grouchy individual.

At times you may think that the person is acting this way because he wants to get back at you for something you did or did not do, or you may think he is trying to be mean to get out of doing something asked of him. It is possible that the person is consciously being irritable in order to manipulate you, but it is not probable. Due to damage to the person's filtering system, he is not able to block out excessive noises. Due to cognitive or thinking deficits, he cannot always figure out why certain happenings are necessary. Due to memory problems, he may not remember that he just told you thirty minutes ago that he did not want Aunt Susan to come over. All of these issues are related to damage to the brain and can lead to a short-tempered, irritable individual.

EXAMPLES

1. Nothing at home seems to please your loved one - he complains about everything.
2. His friends come around less and less, telling you that they find him difficult to get along with.
3. He finds it difficult to allow others to listen to T.V. because the noise is annoying to him.
4. He always has critical things to say about your friends.
5. He becomes very anxious and agitated when he has to go see his physician.

RESOLUTIONS

1. It is useless to say "Why are you so grouchy!" He probably does not understand or even realize the magnitude of his personality change.
2. If there are certain people that your loved one finds irritating, then minimize the time that is spent with those individuals when possible.
3. Provide whatever comfort is needed when the person becomes agitated - often he just needs a reassuring remark or pat on the back to reduce the agitation.
4. Keep surprises and changes to a minimum - individuals who are brain injured do not react positively to either of these.
5. Allow the person to talk through his problems - this can reduce the agitation, but you might listen over and over to the same topic.
6. Keep loud and intrusive noises to a minimum.
7. Develop methods of compromising. You should not give in entirely to the patient, but it may be necessary to make allowances.
8. Do not take the irritability personally - it is not you that is causing the bad mood.

9. If you feel that your loved one has begun to use his irritability in order to get his way, make sure that you do not allow this type of manipulation. You may need some assistance from a therapist or counselor to turn this habit around.

B. OUTBURSTS: ACT BEFORE THINKING

With a short fuse, the person who is brain injured can display a multitude of physical and/or verbal outbursts. Excessive swearing is a common characteristic, and one that can be most embarrassing to family members. Often an individual who is brain injured will blurt out something that he is admittedly sorry for later, yet he continues to do this with little change in his behavior no matter how badly he says he feels each and every time it happens.

Although it is common for individuals who are brain injured to become physically abusive, this does not mean that your family should have to live in terror of this abuse. There are brain injury facilities that are specifically set up to deal with these types of serious behavior problems. Your loved one may need to go to one of these special centers in order to bring this behavior under control. If the individual comes home and you find the physical assaults are unmanageable, explore the possibility of a behavioral center.

The reality is that you will need to make some allowances or concessions for the fact that this individual will often act before he thinks, not unlike the small child who has to be trained to take many things into consideration before he sets his mouth or body into motion. You will need to retrain some of these social skills in order to assist your loved one in becoming an accepted member of society again. This is no small job. Use all the professional resources you can find to assist you.

EXAMPLES

1. You are shocked at the bad language. Prior to the accident you had rarely heard your loved one swear. Now it is a daily occurrence.
2. Your husband gets physically abusive when he had never lifted a finger in your direction before the accident.
3. The adolescent who is brain injured threatens to kill his teacher.
4. The student who is brain injured becomes a significant behavior problem at school. Before the accident he had never been to the principal's office for discipline.
5. The once mild and complacent husband tells his mother-in-law to "butt out or go home."
6. Your husband pulls the phone out of the wall after his daughter's boyfriend calls for the third time that night.

RESOLUTIONS

1. In reference to swearing, try to ignore it as much as possible. If he thinks this is terribly annoying to you, it could increase in frequency as he tries to get your attention.
2. Let him know that verbal abuse or screaming is not the best way for him to get his needs met by not meeting them when he acts this way. For example, "I will not listen to you when you scream at me," or "If you would like to ask that another way, we can discuss it," or "I will not stay in the room when you talk to me that way."
3. Teach the individual the skill of stopping and thinking before he speaks. You can devise a signal (holding up 2 fingers or crossed fingers or whatever sign you want) in order to get the person to consider carefully what he is going to say. This silent signal

is effective in public because it does not have to look like you are treating him like a child. Other signals could be as follows:

a. squeezing your nose

b. scratching your head

c. winking

4. Talk to friends and neighbors and explain to them about these brain injury behaviors. Do this before the individual comes home rather than after he has blown off steam at someone. Tell people not to take the verbiage personally or to react to physical threats. In most cases these will be just that - threats.

5. Learn to build a thick coating around any sensitive feelings you have. Personal sensitivity is a trait that is counterproductive to living with an individual who is brain injured.

6. Do not badger the person about past verbal or physical transgressions - it won't help.

7. Do not allow yourself to live under physical abuse - get professional help.

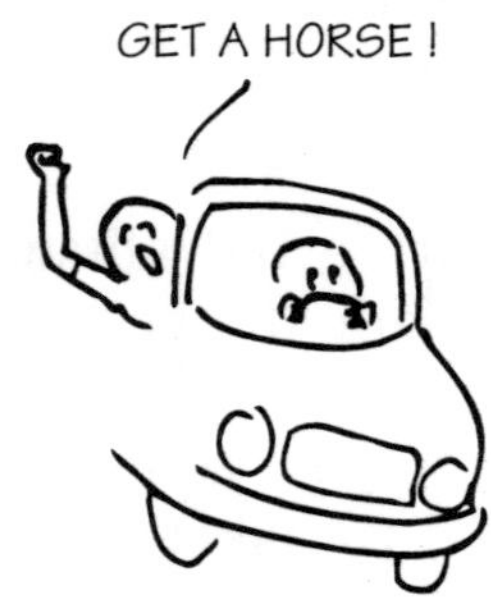

C. FAMILY ABUSE

The behaviors previously addressed, as well as others yet to be covered, all impact upon what is probably the greatest deterrent to a family continuing to provide long-term support for the individual who is brain injured. This is out and out family abuse. Many of us were raised to believe that we should stand by our family members through thick and thin. Putting up with brain injury behaviors can definitely qualify as a challenge to this type of commitment.

One of the most aggravating things that families experience is that, when the rehab nurse or someone like this comes to visit, your loved one who is brain injured can be the picture of politeness. Once you see that he can act appropriately, it is more difficult to accept the abusive behavior that is dished out on a regular basis. There are many different explanations for this, none of which makes it any easier to tolerate, but they do provide a framework for understanding.

First of all, we all tend to let our hair down with family as opposed to strangers or acquaintances. Of course an injured person's loved one's interpretation of "hair down" usually goes beyond what you or I would consider acceptable. They are used to saying whatever they think to their family knowing that this is not a problem. However, after a brain injury there is the added openness and abrasiveness that are new to family members.

Secondly, the individual who is brain injured often loses some of his social judgment capabilities and is not able to effectively reason out behavior or the behavior he expects from others.

All in all, a family's patience can be worn quite thin over months and months of care of this individual. What makes matters worse is that the person who is brain injured has little insight into the impact that he is having on the family.

EXAMPLES

1. The adolescent spits in his mother's face when she says he is not allowed to drive the car yet.
2. The grandfather screams constantly at the young grand-children he adored and spoiled prior to his accident.
3. The husband constantly accuses his wife of cheating on him.
4. The woman slaps her 60 year old mother as she tries to help her into the shower.
5. The man who is brain injured does not allow his daughter's boyfriend to come in the house, saying he is not good enough for his daughter. Therefore, she has to sneak around and go out with him without her father knowing. Even though he did not particularly like the boy prior to his accident, he kept most of his thoughts to himself.

RESOLUTIONS

1. Do not allow a pattern of family abuse to become established in your home upon discharge. Yes, you will need to make some allowances, but continued abuse is not acceptable.
2. Do not continually bring up reminders of his abusive behavior. This will only serve to upset him and will not be conducive to change.
3. There should be family rules that the person is aware of prior to coming home. It is much better to present them ahead of time rather than setting them up once a person has broken some unwritten rule.
4. Get all family members together before discharge and set up consistent methods that will be used by everyone in handling and interacting with the individual. You should ask the therapists to provide

you with management techniques that have worked at the rehab facility.

5. Never allow yourself to get into the "push-me, pull-you" struggle. It is almost impossible to win an argument with a person who is brain injured, because they are almost always convinced they are correct - so don't get into this no win trap.

6. It is very important that the young children of a parent who is brain injured be provided with counseling and assistance in understanding their parent's problems, so that they will not feel personally responsible for difficulties that arise.

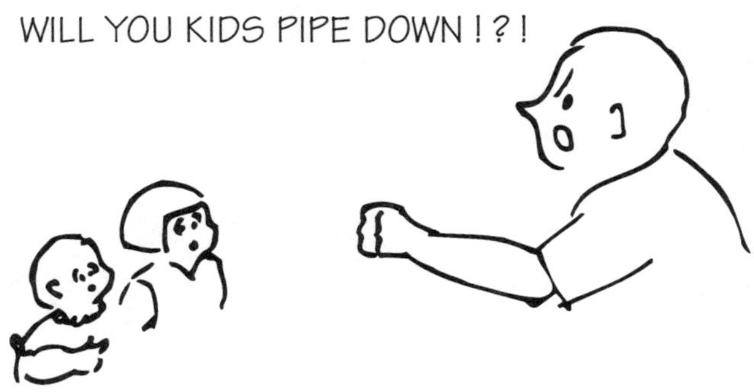

D. ME, ME, ME

One of the reasons why the individual who is brain injured continues to add to family abuse is the completely self-centered approach he often takes to life. The world revolves around him and his problems.

To some degree it is true that no family member completely comprehends what the injured person is experiencing. Nevertheless, this is no excuse for insisting that his needs be put above all others. Your loved one will have to relearn the reality that the world is made up of many other people, and their wishes and desires are also important. This job falls upon you since you are going to be the one to help him reintegrate into the community. He may need to be told in many different ways that the world does not center around him.

EXAMPLES

1. The individual constantly complains, "You don't know what it is like to have a brain injury."
2. The husband does not understand why his working wife does not have supper ready right at 6:00 p.m. when she gets off work at 5:00 p.m.
3. The parent who is brain injured finds himself in competition with his children for the attention and time of his spouse.
4. The injured individual believes that his rehab nurse wants him to get therapy so that he will not have time to go back to work.
5. The individual believes that there should be a family member ready to take him where he needs to go at a moment's notice.

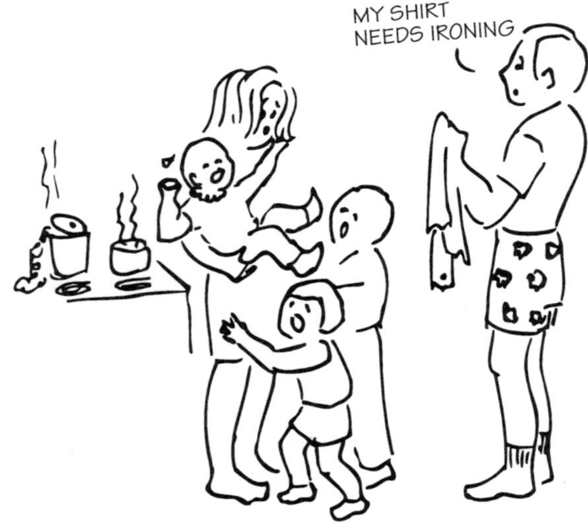

RESOLUTIONS

1. Do not let your whole family schedule center around the injured individual. Let him know that his needs are important, but so are the needs of other family members.

2. Do not allow the patient to put you on a guilt trip.
3. Help the person try to understand the other people's point of view. Sometimes he has to be guided to put himself in another person's place.
4. Help him realize that people outside of the family will look negatively upon him if he acts self-centered.
5. Participation in a brain injury support group often helps the person focus on other people's problems and not just on his own.

E. DEPENDENCY

The role of rehabilitation is to help the individual who is brain injured become as independent as possible. Thus, it is very important that upon discharge you know exactly what he can do for himself. The minute you start to give in and do things for him you will begin to undermine weeks and months of rehabilitation efforts. We all enjoy being waited on at times and you may feel that you want to show the person that you love him, but, doing things that he can do is not the way to show this love.

Individuals who are brain injured also become very dependent on others in making important decisions. If it is not a critical issue where you need to help the person come to the "right" conclusion, force him to decide and accept whatever he chooses. You might also set up decision opportunities in the family structure so that he will have a chance to practice his decision making skills.

EXAMPLES

1. The individual who is brain injured will discuss the same issue over and over with the social worker, then the psychologist, then the therapist, then the neighbor, etc., etc., etc. And even after all this time he may not have made a decision about the issue.

2. The adolescent expects that his best friend will do everything with him and, if he does not, he will not go out with anybody else.
3. He expects his wife to make all the calls to cancel therapy when he is not going to go that day.
4. He has his mother make all the contacts with his rehabilitation nurse.

RESOLUTIONS

1. Allow the individual to make as many of his own decisions as possible.
2. Refuse to tell him what to do unless it is absolutely necessary.
3. Encourage outings with people outside the family.
4. Do not allow yourself to be overprotective.
5. Become active in a supportive group - maybe the individual will find someone else to help rather than concentrate on being helped.

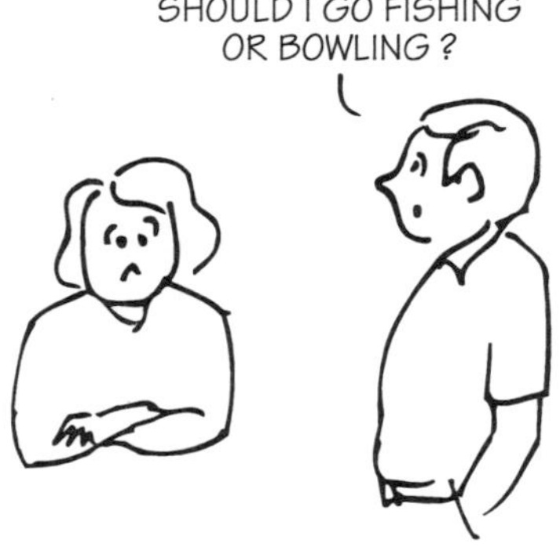

F. DENIAL

From the time your injured loved one could talk again, you have probably noticed that he is not always realistic about what he is capable of doing. This is a characteristic that often lasts a lifetime to some degree. In the field of rehabilitation we call it denial. At first this denial is beneficial because it keeps the individual motivated. However, as time goes on it can lead to anger and depression. The anger occurs because the individual is convinced that he should be able to go back to work and that people are unjustifiably keeping him from this. You may have heard your loved one enumerate a long list of people who are at fault for his lack of progress and/or impede his return to the real world.

It is a delicate proposition to balance the protective quality of denial and the rehabilitative need for reality. It usually is not necessary to take away all hope of living independently, going back to work, getting married, etc. The best way to handle these issues upon discharge is to indicate that there are a number of steps that the individual must go through before those goals are obtainable. For example, if you are getting bugged daily about your son wanting to live in his house that he owns, let him know that the steps are as follows:

1) Possibly live in a transitional living facility where additional skills will be mastered.

2) Move to supervised apartments until minimal supervision is needed.

3) Move back into your home with support of family, friends, or hired aide.

The reality may be that you and the therapists are thinking that the end goal is not feasible. However, keep focusing on the fact that he still has steps 1, 2, and 3 to work toward.

EXAMPLES

1. The man is convinced that his wife is willing and ready to take care of him even though she has filed for divorce.

2. The woman is sure that her boss at the law firm will take her back as a legal secretary.

3. The adolescent says that his Dad has a new truck ready to replace the one he wrecked just as soon as he gets out of the wheelchair.

4. The parents refuse to talk about appropriate special education placement or assistance as they are sure their daughter will be able to return to her regular classrooms.

5. The man does not see any need for a therapist to talk to his employer since he knows he can go back to work and do everything he did before the accident.

HOW MANY TIMES
DO I HAVE TO
DO THIS ?
TILL YOU CAN
DO IT RIGHT
OT

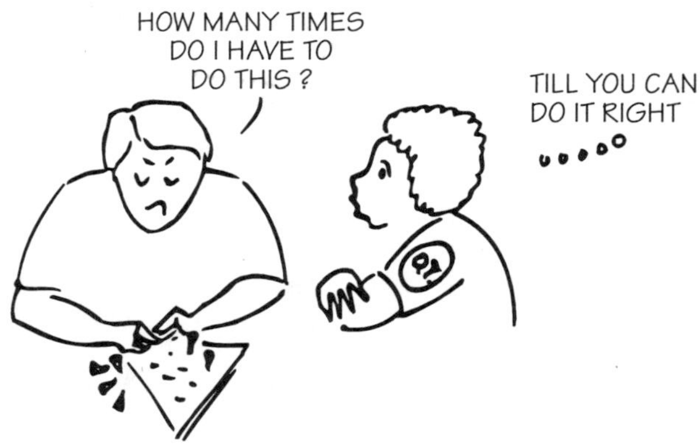

RESOLUTIONS

1. Allow the individual to hold onto some denial in order to maintain his motivation to participate in rehabilitation.

2. Never out and out lie to your loved one, saying he will be able to do something that seems unlikely. Instead, point out the progress that is necessary to get to that particular goal.

3. If the person who is brain injured insists he can do something and it would not be dangerous to him or anyone else, allow him to try the activity. This can often lead to a realization that he is not quite ready to complete this task on his own.

4. If your loved one tries to tell you that he is not getting anything out of occupational therapy because he is always doing the same things, do not be coerced into thinking that the therapist does not have anything else for him to do. The reason he is repeating tasks is that he has not completed them correctly or with the desired speed - he needs more practice.

5. It is important for you to know that at times when your loved one is being obstinate and refusing to cooperate, this may be his way of avoiding (denying) facing the fact that the activity is too difficult for him. He may see that it should be simple and not want to face the reality that he cannot do something that simple.

6. Participation in a brain injury support group is often a good place for the individual to hear other people talk about their difficulties and how they have dealt with them. This can make it a little easier for him to identify and admit to his own deficits.

G. SUSPICIOUSNESS

Individuals who are brain injured often have difficulty drawing appropriate conclusions about social situations. As a result, he can persist in paranoid type behavior and thinking that bears little resemblance to reality. This can be very disconcerting to family members who are putting everything they have into helping this individual and are getting unjustly accused of wrongful deeds.

The best way to handle this is to try to separate yourself from the false accusations - do not allow them to get you down. You can say something such as "It disappoints me when you talk this way," or "It makes me sad to hear you say such things." Then walk away and try not to dwell upon the issue. You will only succeed in upsetting yourself more.

EXAMPLES

1. The husband interprets every call where a person hangs up as some other man calling for his wife.
2. The son accuses his mother of not allowing him to regain his competency because she wants to steal his money.
3. The adolescent is convinced that his best friend is turning his girlfriend against him.
4. The individual believes that the only reason he is not back to work is that his therapist called up his boss and told him he could not do the job anymore.
5. Your son insists that you are giving away some of his clothes that he cannot find (they are actually stuffed under his bed where he put them while cleaning his room).

RESOLUTIONS

1. Do not argue about the suspicious thoughts. You will never convince him otherwise through verbal argument.
2. The best stance to take is to ignore, ignore, ignore.
3. Never show your anger - he will interpret this as an admission of guilt.
4. If there is a therapist involved with the individual, ask him to help you work through the issue that is of particular concern to the loved one who is brain injured. Sometimes all of you talking together will alleviate the concern.
5. It is possible that the injured one should talk to a therapist about his suspicious thoughts. If not alleviated, these thoughts can eat at him and lead to greater problems in other areas.
6. If you think your loved one can handle it, it might do good to have the object of his suspicions confront him. For example, if he is accusing the male nurse

of having "eyes" for you, have the nurse sit down with him and discuss the issue. This stance can be very effective. However, it can backfire, so proceed with caution.

7. Try to guide your family member's thinking in a more positive direction.

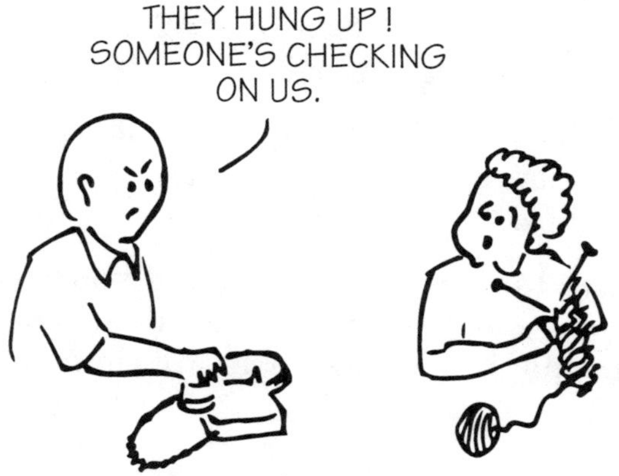

H. PERSEVERATION

The definition of perseveration is talking about something over and over, or obsessing on an action or idea over and over. Brain injury entails two main characteristics that lead to this type of behavior. First, difficulty with short-term memory leads to the individual having little to no recognition that he has discussed this issue no less than a half hour before. Moreover, the cognitive problems related to inadequate problem solving skills lead the individual who is brain injured into the necessity of rehashing issues incessantly, so that they are never adequately resolved or solved by the person himself.

As a result, you will more than likely have three to four recurring themes or conversations that occur over and over until you will think you are going to scream. It may be next to impossible to change this behavior entirely, but there are some ways you can learn to live with it and tolerate it.

EXAMPLES

1. Your husband who is brain injured talks constantly about your daughter's terrible husband.
2. Your son speaks daily of getting his driver's license renewed.
3. The husband continually writes letters to his vocational rehabilitation counselor stating that he is not being properly helped.
4. The neighbor's dog is a continual subject of conversation each time there is evidence it has been in your yard.
5. Your loved one tells every one of your friends a long drawn out story about his accident, even when the same people have heard it many times before.

RESOLUTIONS

1. If there is some burning issue upon which the individual dwells, set up a designated time for discussing that issue each day. Then do not participate in any conversation regarding it except at the specific time. For instance, tell your loved one that the issue of his returning to his job will be discussed only from 5:30 to 6:00 p.m. each day.
2. If the issue is something that is definitely not feasible or is unsolvable at this time, you can refuse to engage in any type of conversation until it becomes a viable alternative. For example, tell your loved one that talking about him living on his own right now is non-productive until he can demonstrate that he can care for himself in specific areas.
3. Be firm and say that you refuse to discuss the same topic any more. If he continues, walk away. Do not feel badly about being very up-front with the person. Sometimes the social amenities we use with others

are too subtle for the individual who is brain injured to process.

4. Try to divert the conversation to another topic. Oftentimes it is easy to lead him into another train of thought.

5. Constant talking about an area of concern is, of course, a sign of anxiety. In many ways the talking is therapeutic (to a point). Take what you can tolerate, and then divert the individual to another subject.

6. Remember, you may think you are doing the loved one a favor by listening over and over; however, in the long run this may not be the case. When he is constantly talking about a worrisome issue he is physically experiencing anxiety. We all know that stress and anxiety can have a negative effect on one's physical health. Thus, you are actually doing him a favor by minimizing the time he obsesses on the issue.

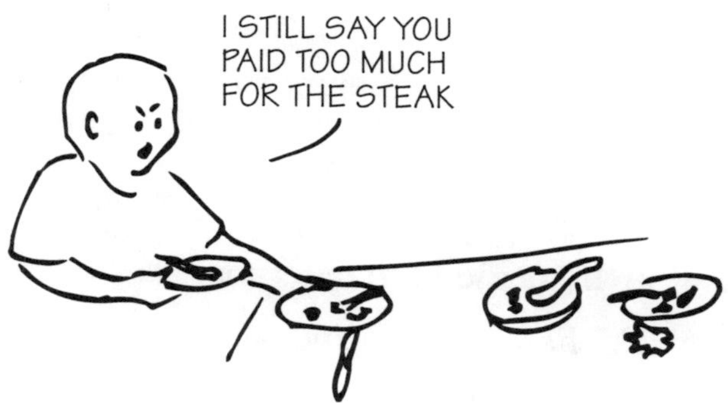

I. DEPRESSION

It seems unusual to think of any emotional state, and particularly depression, as a sign of progress. However, in the field of brain injury rehabilitation the occurrence of a depressed state indicates that the individual is giving up some of that denial that is often counterproductive to progress. It is important for the person to realize that he does in fact have deficits, and that these deficits will have an impact upon his future.

In spite of the positive effects of letting go of some denial, the same safeguards apply regarding an individual experiencing a depressive state. Once you recognize the fact that your loved one is depressed, you must be able to walk the fine line between keeping him motivated and helping him to realistically modify his goals.

EXAMPLES

1. Your loved one is difficult to get up and about in the morning (a change from previous patterns). He sleeps ten or more hours at night and naps in the day.
2. You note a change in eating habits - either a noticeable reduction or increase in consumption.
3. Remarks regarding the futility of going on, such as "What's the sense in all of this, " or "It would be better if I had been killed in the accident" are signs of this state.
4. Your loved one may begin to remember the past with greater frequency, durations, and emotional labeling.
5. A person who was not an avid T.V. fan now spends hour after hour glued to the tube.
6. His "spark" has disappeared.

RESOLUTIONS

1. Take all expressions of suicidal thoughts and plans seriously - seek professional assistance and guidance.
2. Do not allow the individual to vegetate - get him out and about as best you can.

3. Do not allow the person to make you feel that you are the cause of the depression. He probably knows better. Even so, do not accept the guilt.

4. If the depression is extremely severe, consult a physician familiar with brain injury regarding the possibility of medication.

5. Do not allow yourself to get down, too.

6. Do not become too overprotective once you have obtained professional help.

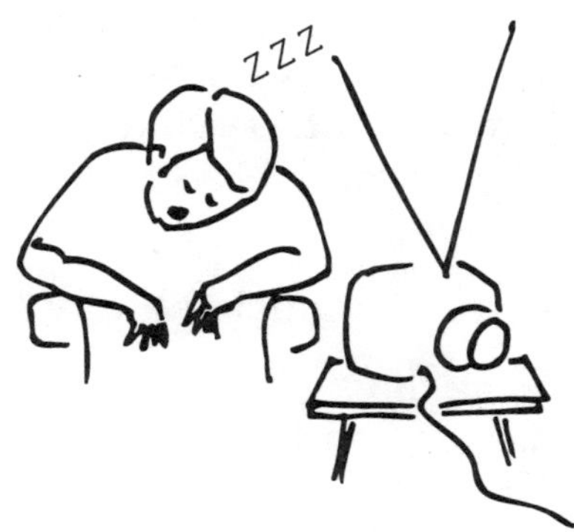

J. LACK OF MOTIVATION / INITIATION

Have members of your family accused your loved one who is brain injured of being lazy? Do they say "If he would only get off his duff and try he could work." Members of the immediate family are usually aware of the reasons for the inertia, but others interpret this "no get-up and go" as the individual's fault.

There are two main issues leading to the reality that this individual looks unmotivated. First, one of the cognitive or thinking deficits related to brain injury is that he has difficulty planning and goal setting. He does not know where or how to start a project so he does not begin.

On top of this, he understands to some degree that he does not have the abilities he had before. Since he does not want to admit to this deficiency, he acts like he is not interested or motivated. The reality is that he is interested but incapable of doing what would have been simple for him before the injury.

EXAMPLES

1. The boss says that all he does is get ready to do the job, but he rarely is able to begin efficiently and follow through.
2. You have asked your loved one to wash a few loads of laundry while you are gone. When you return nothing has been done. He tells you the washing powder was not above the washer on the shelf so he assumed you were out. He had not looked on the floor beside the dryer where there was a large box ready to be opened.
3. He sits and listens to music all day long.
4. The therapist is having a difficult time finding a reinforcer that is powerful enough to keep him activated in therapy.
5. The loved one who is brain injured uses very flimsy excuses to get out of going to therapy.
6. He shows little interest in a baseball card collection that was his avid hobby prior to the brain injury.
7. He makes adequate plans and promises, but he has great difficulty following through.

RESOLUTIONS

1. Give the individual who is brain injured the needed supervision to start a task, since you now know that getting started can be the biggest problem.
2. Never assume that, because he did a task perfectly before the injury, he is now being lazy or obstinate if he does not complete it.

3. If he asks for help on an activity never assume that he does not need it. In fact, assume he does need help until he completes it on his own.
4. If possible, break tasks down into smaller parts so that he can easily understand, remember, and master them.
5. You may need to get help from a professional to set up a management program to break an inactivity cycle.
6. If your loved one has been excessively agitated for an extended period of time, do not breathe a sigh of relief once he becomes inert. Although this is much more relaxing for you, it is not better for your loved one.
7. Never ask questions such as "Do you want to. . . " There is too much opportunity to say "No" and remain passive. Give choices of two or three activities whereby the family member must agree to choose one.
8. Get your loved one involved in a support group. This will be at least one activity a month, or maybe even twice a month depending on the group.
9. If you have the energy and time, offer your house as a place for patients who are brain injured and their families to meet and engage in social activities.

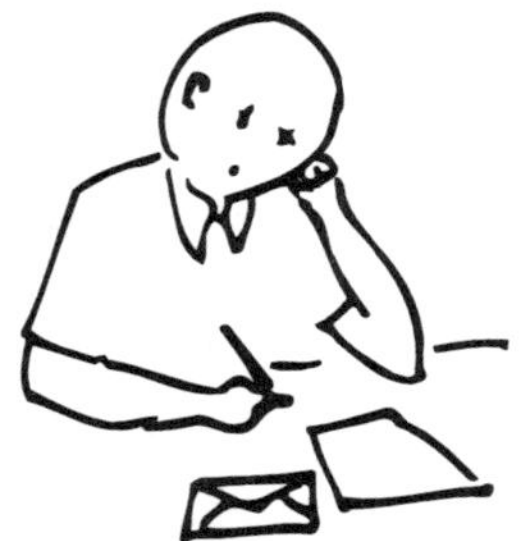

K. SOCIAL IMMATURITY

For a loved one who cannot be recognized as a person with a brain injury from outward appearances, it is sometimes the inappropriate social interactions that give him away. There are many reasons for the presence of this deficit. The first, of course, involves cognitive issues, whereby the individual does not completely understand what is going on but joins in the conversation. The fact that his topic is unrelated is a sure sign that he falls into a handicapped category.

Another area that relates to this is the recently described area of egocentricism. Everything said is interpreted from the injured one's viewpoint so that there are few empathetic responses - only egocentric responses. The individual who is brain injured may be able to turn this around, to some degree, but the turn can be too sharp. He may go from talking only about himself to asking somebody how much money he makes.

The subtleties of social situations are lost. The person must be retrained to think before he acts or talks. He will need to learn to censor or revamp his interactions depending upon the audience. The skill is an advanced one and may need the help of a therapist if you have the means and availability in your area.

EXAMPLES

1. Your family member asks the cashier at the grocery store if she is married.

2. He tells the teller at the bank that he talks this way because he had a brain injury and proceeds to tell her about the accident.
3. The individual who is brain injured, in a support group of family and peers, starts to tell about some inappropriate activities a person took toward him the night before.
4. He becomes very upset when the family decides, due to financial considerations, to go to McDonald's instead of a more expensive restaurant.
5. He does not understand why his aunt cannot take him to the mall as she promised. The explanation that she has come down with the flu is not adequate.

RESOLUTIONS

1. You will need to retrain your loved one to act in a socially appropriate manner.
2. Do not get discouraged. Social skills are not acquired overnight.
3. When you get ready to go out, remind your loved one that he is not to talk to strangers about personal matters.
4. Devise a signal whereby you call his name and proceed with some kind of nonverbal cue such as scratching your nose, licking your lips, or clearing your throat. He should be taught that the signal means that it is not the time or the place to be discussing the subject matter.
5. Do not reinforce inappropriate behavior by acting angry - he may continue to bring a subject up because he sees it upsets you.
6. Remember that bringing the person who is brain injured back home is like starting all over again in helping him to relearn normal social behavior.

WHADDA YA PULL DOWN ON
A JOB LIKE THIS ?
SERVICE

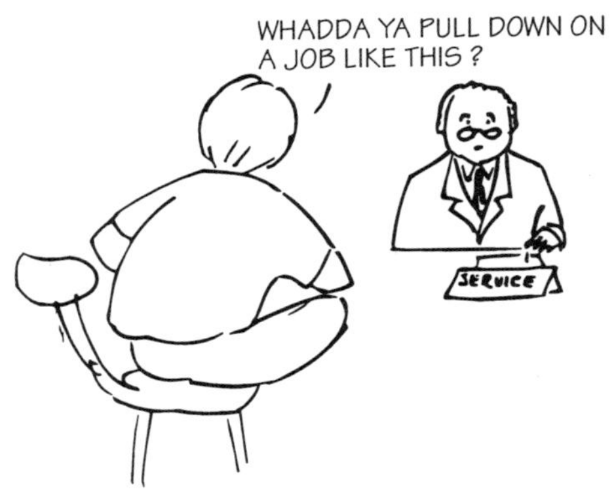

L. INCREASED SEXUAL OPENNESS

An individual's sexual orientation and activity can be modified by a blow to the head. In some cases the area of the brain that regenerates various hormones can be thrown off. In other words, the injured person's ability to inhibit can be altered. Some people who are brain injured turn away or reject sexual activity. However, others may turn a major focus upon remarks, actions, innuendoes, or anything remotely related to the subject of sex.

For those of you who have had a fairly conservative family upbringing in relation to sex, this change can be very difficult. You are not used to such comments, jokes, or overtures that can become daily occurrences in this person's life. You are not equipped to hear or see these things, much less to learn to modify the responses.

I BET YOU'RE CUTE
WITH YOUR HAIR DOWN

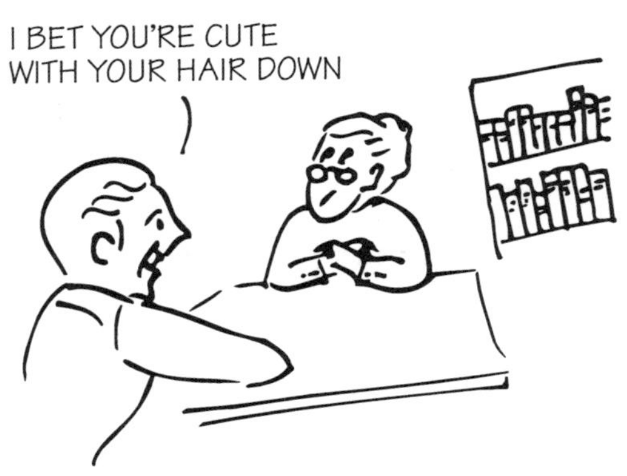

Social contacts of your family and the person with a brain injury will turn away from your loved one because they are uncomfortable in his company. They will be hard pressed to understand why he is making a pass at their girlfriend or wife. The result, of course, will be social isolation. Once this occurs, the injured person begins to blame others for the isolation. He has a difficult time understanding how his remarks have been offensive.

We realize that this remains a major difficulty with many individuals who are brain injured. We have seen cases where there was an increase in sexual obsession four or more years after the injury. The avid interest is predictable, but the manner of expression, intensity, and duration differs from individual to individual.

EXAMPLES

1. The patient has scared off every attendant due to sexual advances.
2. He has been arrested or threatened with arrest due to showing private parts in public.
3. He takes every opportunity to grab or touch other people.
4. He takes a very assertive approach which tends to scare people off.
5. He talks constantly about wanting to marry.
6. He refuses to allow anyone over 40 or of the wrong sex to be his therapist or attendant.
7. The husband becomes very angry and threatening when the wife does not desire sexual intimacy at a particular time.

RESOLUTIONS

1. Each time the individual behaves inappropriately a designated family member should tell him, in a

nonthreatening and noncombative manner, that the behavior is unacceptable.

2. Therapist and attendants should, as much as possible, position themselves so that they are not within arm's reach.
3. One should never bother with excess verbiage such as "I am a married woman," "Joe and I are happily married," or "I will tell your mother."
4. Never lecture about the moralistic factors of his behavior. It may make you feel better, but it will have little impact on behavioral change.
5. Consult a sex therapist who has experience working with individuals who are brain injured in your area. If there is no one in the vicinity, you might consult with the Masters and Johnson Institute in St. Louis, Missouri.
6. Keep cool and do not overreact.

M. OVEREATING

Although this does not occur with every person with a brain injury, it is common enough to warrant a note of caution. Underneath the cortex of the brain are areas that deal with hunger, sexual arousal, emotional reactions, etc. Sometimes these areas are damaged, resulting in an inability to determine if you have been satisfied by intake of food. If this occurs, your loved one will appear to have an insatiable appetite - continually eating everything in sight.

While he was in the rehabilitation facility this intake of food was monitored to some degree, depending upon the level of independence available in the center. However, his monitoring will be much more difficult to maintain once your loved one comes home (or even if he's just coming to visit for awhile). We all know that eating is a pleasurable experience. It, therefore, becomes very difficult to deprive him of this pleasure, since you may be thinking that there are too few aspects of his life that are positive these days. Moreover, if you are a mother or father who enjoys cooking, you will find it rewarding to see him delighted by eating some of his favorite meals.

However, do not trade short-term pleasure for long-term health problems. Being overweight is good for no one, but it is particularly devastating to the injured individual's appearance, self-concept, motivation, and "get-up-and-go." So, before this becomes a problem at home that you have to change, get ready to structure low calorie meals with a minimum availability of snacks. You and your loved one will benefit by this regime.

EXAMPLES

1. The loved one buys his favorite peanut butter cups every time he gets a chance.
2. You find that the entire dozen doughnuts are gone within a few hours of your returning from the store.
3. He wishes that you feel guilty because you do not make his favorite cake every weekend.
4. You find candy bars hoarded away in his underwear drawer.

RESOLUTIONS

1. Do not equate eating with a healthy body. By this time he does not require those extra calories he needed when he was in an acute care setting.
2. Do not buy fattening foods - it is much easier to have them unavailable than to ration them out.
3. Model good eating habits yourself.
4. Initiate a daily weigh-in system (you too!), so that the weight will not get out of hand before you notice. It is much easier to initially avoid food than to diet to lose.

5. If things are already out of control, consider a regimented program such as Weight Watchers or Nutri-System.

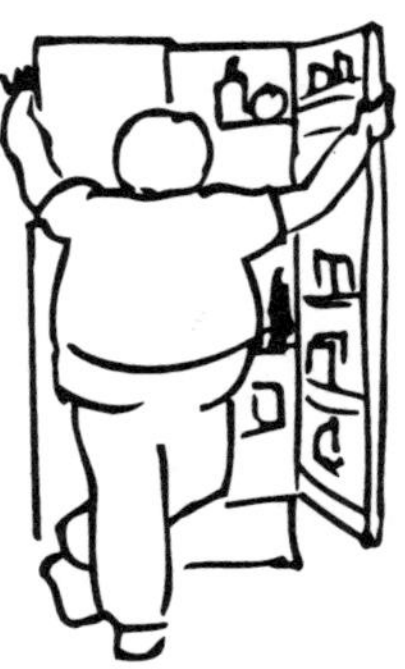

IX. FAMILY BEHAVIORS

For those of you who have already lived with an individual who is brain injured, you are well aware of the emotional reactions that you experienced. There is no question but that bringing your loved one home changes your life and impacts upon your mental health status. The purpose of this section is to prepare these responses for you to use, as well as letting you know that it is not wrong, unusual, or immature of you to think or do some of the things discussed in this section.

Even the average run of the mill family (if such a family exists) has problems that they face each day. Many of these problems are understood and recognized by middle-class America. However, living with an individual who is brain injured is not one bit like "The Brady Bunch," "All In The Family," or "Family Ties." It is a different world that only those who have experienced it or worked with those who are going through it can understand. It is often helpful to find a support group in your community to attend and share some of your problems. If there is not one around and you have the time and energy, you might consider starting one. You can contact a local hospital or church for a meeting space. You can obtain assistance and ideas from the Brain Injury Association for additional ways of contacting others in your area.

A. ANXIETY

You probably are familiar with the state of excessive worries and fears that can occur within families of individuals who are brain injured, unless you are indeed different from most families who have lived through the trauma. My guess is that you are no exception. While your loved one remains under medical and rehabilitation care, there are many things to cause you anxious feelings: What will life be like for him? Will he be able to raise his family? Will he be able to support himself? Is he getting the right type of therapy? Is he getting enough therapy?

As extensive as these concerns can be, they are never as all encompassing as the day to day worries of having the person return to your home. Now you can worry about all the things mentioned before, as well as a multitude of additional concerns: Is he sleeping too much? Why won't he come out of his room? Is he constipated? Are the medications causing his lethargy? Why do his friends not come to visit? Why is his wife keeping the children away? Why does he get so mad at me? If necessary, we could produce three to four pages of these fears and anxieties and there would still be others your family members could include.

Once you know that your loved one is being discharged, start to prepare yourself to accept the fact that there will be problem areas. You will approach each in a logical manner, do what you can with the knowledge you possess, get help from those who can assist, and promise not to make an obsession of those things that are out of your control.

EXAMPLES

1. You are concerned about whether his wife will be able to accept his deficiencies.

2. You worry that there will not be enough money or adequate insurance to handle his life-long care.

3. You wonder if the doctor was correct when you were told he would never go back to work.
4. You are not sure what is meant by "adequate supervision."
5. You think that his depression is interfering with him reintegrating himself back into the community.

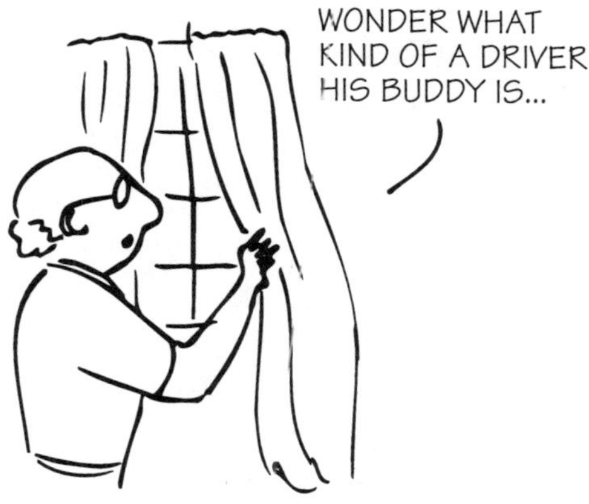

RESOLUTIONS

1. Schedule your times to think about worrying subjects, such as between 8:00 and 9:00 a.m. Then forbid yourself to obsess or concentrate on your many concerns the rest of the day.
2. If your family member who is brain injured is engaged in constant verbalization about a concern of his, do <u>not</u> allow yourself to get trapped into worrying constantly with him. One person worrying at a time is enough.
3. Remember that excess worrying is bad for your health.
4. If you find yourself going "over the edge," contact a mental health professional.
5. Remember that your worries should not control your life. You should control your life - you should control your worries.

6. Participate in a support group for brain injury. Many of them will have already resolved some of the worries that are new to you. There is nothing like the voice of experience.

B. OVEROPTIMISM

Optimism is a powerful force to keep you through times when hard core pessimists might give up. However, there is a fine line between the positive effect of optimism and the negative effect of overoptimism. We all want to believe that our loved one will get better - but, it is very often not wise to assume that he will completely return to his original capabilities.

There are various ways in which this can be counterproductive. First, your family member is now being discharged from a rehabilitation facility. Before he entered the facility you had some expectations about what could be accomplished while he was there. Now he is leaving the program and he may not have attained all the skills you expected. There are two different types of negative approaches that you can take. You can say that the rehabilitation facility was not adequate and, therefore, did not do what needed to be done. Or you can say that your loved one was not cooperative or motivated enough to profit from what the center had to offer. In the first instance you may find yourself going from facility to facility looking for the place that can accomplish what you think is feasible. In the second instance, your loved one will assume that he is entirely at fault.

If at all possible, it is best for you to take the recovery period a day at a time without planning too far ahead. In essence, the right mixture is a nice amount of optimism tempered with a touch of realism.

EXAMPLES

1. You have told his old boss that he will be ready to come back to work after he is discharged from the center.

2. His wife is expecting that his personality changes will be gone, or at least considerably diminished.
3. You feel that all has been a failure if he is not walking independently at discharge.
4. You have told your loved one who is brain injured that he can do anything if he just tries hard enough.

RESOLUTIONS

1. One day at a time - make that your motto.
2. Do not make the loved one feel that he has failed if he has not met your expectations.
3. Remember, people can live productive lives from a wheelchair.
4. Try to make him feel as if he is worthwhile, even with the current limitations.
5. Emphasize all the positive recovery that has occurred.

OH SHE'S ALWAYS BEEN AN HONOR STUDENT. I'M SURE SHE'LL HAVE NO TROUBLE.

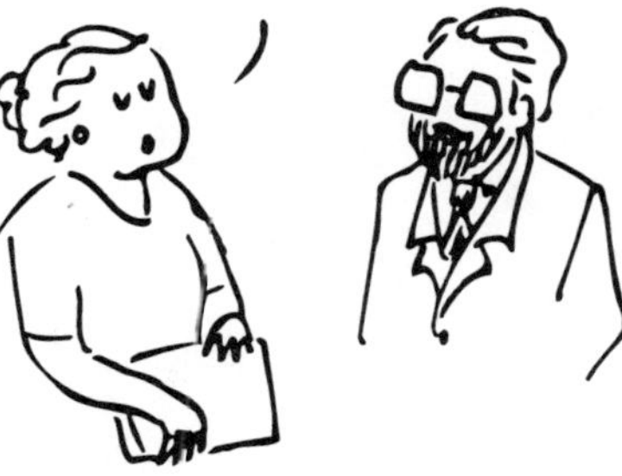

C. FRUSTRATION

Frustration is an emotional reaction you experience that is present from the time of the injury through your loved one's lifetime. The focus and intensity changes, but the presence of frustrating experiences is a given. While in the rehabilitation facility you may have been frustrated by what you saw as a lack of communication, agency red-tape, frustration with case management, and problems with the funding source, to mention just a few possible areas.

Now that your loved one is ready to be discharged, you will run into all the drawbacks of attempting to reintegrate him into the community. The reality of how prepared society is to accept and help those individuals is upon you.

EXAMPLES

1. Your physician says that he will not authorize any further treatment, as your loved one is at Maximum Medical Improvement (MMI).
2. Vocational rehabilitation does not see your family member as a feasible candidate.
3. The rehabilitation nurse says that the insurance company will not pay for a day treatment program.
4. You are told that his psychiatric problems are unrelated to the brain injury.
5. His friends are turning away from him and he is becoming more depressed.
6. His employer now says his job is no longer waiting for him.

RESOLUTIONS

1. Frustrations are a reality - it is how you handle them that makes a difference.
2. Never allow yourself to be worked into a frenzy -you will never solve the problems in that state of mind.
3. See if any seminars are being offered in your area on managing and controlling frustration.
4. Remember that the individual who is brain injured will pick up on your frustration and may use this in a negative manner.

5. Speak with others in a support group and find out how they managed their disappointments.
6. Develop alternative methods of reaching your goals for the patient if you find that certain avenues are blocked.

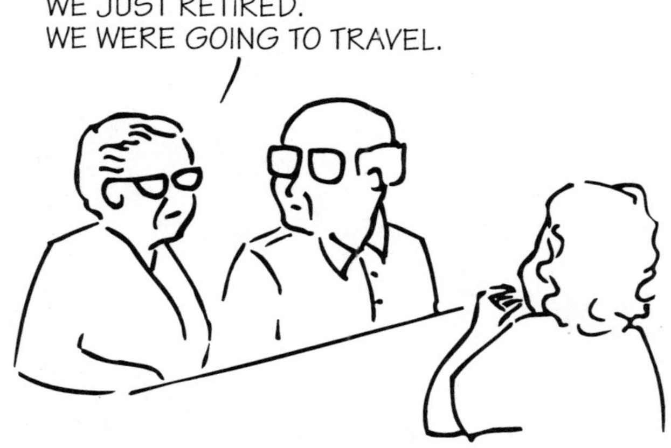

D. EXCESSIVE STRESS

It would be ridiculous to tell you that you should avoid stress. What family with a loved one who is brain injured is without stress? However, here are effective methods of handling your stress and these methods should be put to good use.

Upon discharge, the stress experienced by all family members involved in the individual's rehabilitation will be increased. Not only will your time be more in demand, but your emotional energy will be expended at an increased rate. Again, as is often said throughout this manual, take care of yourself so that you can be "right" for your loved one.

EXAMPLES

1. You are turning into a complete grouch.
2. You find yourself overreacting to minor nuisances (e.g., lost keys, spilled milk, noisy children, excessive telephone calls, etc.).

3. The medical bills are mounting and, with each trip to the mailbox, you become more stressed out.

4. You find it harder and harder to remember things these days - or to keep things straight in your mind.

5. You find that you have a hard time getting to sleep or you wake up at 3:00 and cannot get back to sleep.

RESOLUTIONS

1. Recognize that the patient's behavior is somewhat outside your ultimate control. Do not attempt to change him drastically - some things you alone cannot change.

2. Give yourself some time away so that you can be refreshed and effectively deal with the issues when you are at home.

3. As a family project, enroll in a stress management class offered at the local community mental health center.

4. Whenever high levels of stress result in physical symptoms (e.g., high blood pressure, headaches, anxiety attacks), be sure to see a physician.

5. Stress management books and relaxation training tapes are available at most book stores and would be helpful in learning to manage stress.

6. Delegate and divvy up responsibilities. All family members should pitch in and help - even the individual who is brain injured, if he is capable.

E. IMPATIENCE / IRRITABILITY

Since we all know that irritability can be catching, it stands to reason that your family members can be just as impatient as the injured person himself. Now that discharge is upon you, it is quite likely that your day to day frustration will increase as mentioned earlier. It would be very easy for us to say such things as "Keep up your spirits," "Keep a positive attitude," "Don't let the problems get you down," and on and on. But, we are not going to do that.

The truth is that you will now be faced with an altered lifestyle that is filled with all kinds of justifications for expecting much more than you receive. In fact, you may have to beg, borrow, or steal the little help that you get. We can have minimal impact on all the life stressors, but we can prepare you to understand the situation and attempt some management techniques.

EXAMPLES

1. You think that, if you have to go through another conversation about driving, you will scream.
2. You find that you are much less tolerant toward the children and their "shenanigans."
3. You feel like your life is not your own.
4. You blow up at the rehabilitation nurse, who is really trying to help, but somehow you cannot see that at the time.

RESOLUTIONS

1. Again, "one day at a time" is a great motto.
2. Do not expect agencies to perform in a proficient manner.

3. Do not expect all people to respond to your dilemmas as you would.

4. If you lose your cool with someone you love, take time to apologize.

5. Tell the children that you are under a great deal of pressure and you could use their help rather than their resistance.

6. Prioritize your projects and tackle them one at a time.

F. FAMILY DISCORD

While the individual who is brain injured has been in the rehabilitation facility your family has settled into a certain routine. Now that routine will be turned upside down. Anytime you have a change like this in a family structure there is always the possibility of disunity and imbalance. You may be saying "Oh, it won't be that way with us because we are anxious for him to come home. All of us want him with us."

In spite of the fact that all members feel positive about the discharge, there will still be times when you are at odds with each other. This often happens when family members disagree about what is best for the patient, and the biggest problem is that you both believe you are right. Other difficulties come in when distant family members (aunts, uncles, cousins, nephews) want to tell you what you are doing wrong. It is at this point that you invite them to come care for the individual who is brain injured while you take your trip to the Bahamas - two weeks ought to be plenty of time for them to implement their care plan.

EXAMPLES

1. Aunt Marie thinks that you take your loved one out too much and get him too excited. That is why he is acting out.

2. Uncle George insists that a vegetarian diet is a must to help his memory problems.
3. You find that you are too tired to communicate with your spouse, as you spend night and day planning for your injured son's future.
4. Your husband who is brain injured feels neglected when you spend time with your children.

RESOLUTIONS

1. Before the individual who is brain injured comes home, promise yourselves that you will set aside some time each week to iron out family issues.
2. Never assume everybody loves him and will not resent all the time he needs.
3. Set up an open communication system whereby all family members feel free to constructively communicate their feelings.
4. If family unity seriously deteriorates, then consider counseling to enhance communication and regain a positive family unit.
5. If there were serious problems in the family prior to the injury, you can expect them to remain and possibly elevate. Try to work on these issues prior to the loved one returning home, if possible.

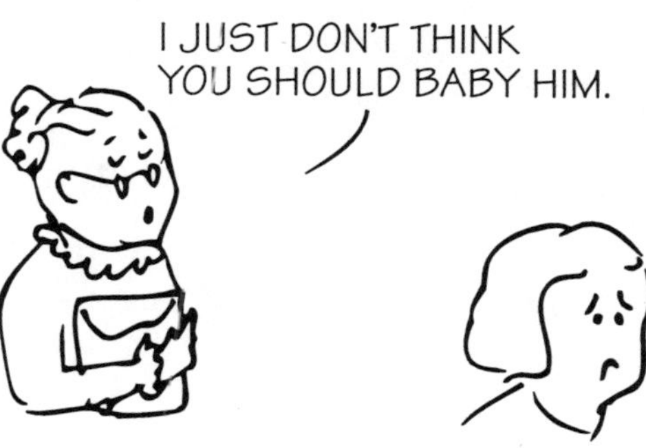

G. DOWN IN THE DUMPS

At this point you may be looking forward to your loved one coming home and, therefore, not be thinking that you might eventually experience depression. On the other hand, if this is the second or third rehabilitation facility, you may well be aware of the letdown that can take place.

It is not unusual for families to experience low points over the course of their loved one's recovery. Remember this when you are at the end of your wits and ready to throw in the towel.

EXAMPLES

1. You feel sleepy all the time and find that you have a hard time getting out of bed.
2. You find that you are drinking more than before.
3. You have a difficult time getting motivated.
4. You are no longer overoptimistic - you have gone in the opposite direction now.
5. Hopeless thoughts occupy your mind.

RESOLUTIONS

1. Take your feelings seriously - seek professional counseling before you find yourself going under.
2. Do not set yourself up for disappointment and depression by assuming or expecting too much.
3. Do not let yourself obsess on negative thoughts.
4. Join a support group where you can voice your concerns to people who really understand.

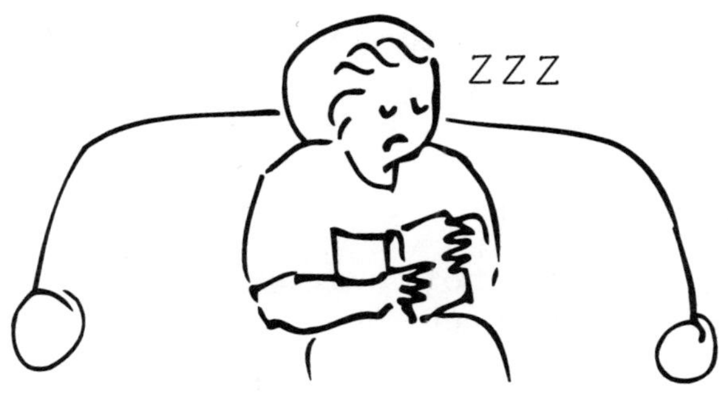

H. GUILT

If you have been a "guilt accumulator" in the past, you will be easily trapped into taking on even greater volumes of guilt now that your loved one is returning home and you are coming face to face with reality. Even if you previously stayed free of guilt, you will have some difficulty avoiding it. The circumstances surrounding living with an individual who is brain injured provide a multitude of possibilities for thinking or feeling that you have not done the best thing in a given situation. Guilt will arise from at least four main sources: 1) you; 2) the loved one; 3) other family members; 4) concerned others. Once you have your own guilt under control, you will have to learn to defuse the guilt laden arrows shot at you by others.

EXAMPLES

1. You may feel guilty every time you go out of the house without your loved one.
2. You may feel guilty that you have not done more to help the individual who is brain injured improve in cognitive skills.
3. You may feel guilty that you have ignored and/or avoided your friends.
4. You may feel guilty that at times you fantasize about a three week vacation alone.

5. You may feel guilty that you have not been able to help the loved one get the vocational training he needs.

RESOLUTIONS

1. Accept guilt as a normal human feeling over which you have minimal control.
2. Substitute some engrossing activity to get your mind off the guilt - gardening, exercising, biking, etc.
3. Schedule your guilt time - only feel guilty on Mondays.
4. Go to a rational - emotive therapist who can help you to quit focusing on what you <u>should</u> have done.

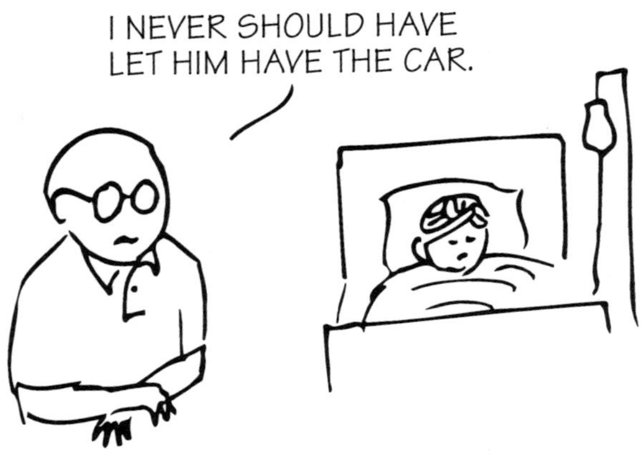

I. SOCIAL ISOLATION

As is often the case when the injured loved one is at home, the family reduces its contact with the outside world to allow their loved one to have a quiet environment and to provide emotional support. The danger there is that this pattern will become a habit that will be hard to break. Studies have shown that the support of family and friends is more important than the assistance of hospital personnel, doctors, or the clergy. Thus, it is a mistake to isolate yourself from your old contacts.

Even though you may make every effort to foster old friendships, you may find that many will gradually drift away due to a variety of reasons: 1) they are not able to understand the injured person's obsession with his physical conditions; 2) they are not able to accept the individual as he presents himself in a group setting; 3) they find that they are uncomfortable in the person's presence because they no longer share common interests and goals. If you find this occurring with a large portion of your former friends, make every effort to form new acquaintances.

EXAMPLES

1. A retired woman takes on the responsibility of her daughter who is brain injured and her three children, and does not make arrangements to see her friends on a social basis.
2. A wife quits her job and gives up outside contacts to attempt to meet all the needs of her husband.
3. The family refuses to go out until the loved one can go to social engagements with them.
4. The husband devotes his entire energy into trying to provide cognitive therapy to his wife. He refuses to go out with his friends from work or to play golf or tennis with his sports companions.
5. A mother gives up her bridge club and discontinues writing letters to her good friends.

RESOLUTIONS

1. Do not set up an early pattern of decreased social contacts.
2. Do not quit your job unless absolutely necessary.
3. When friends call, talk about things other than the patient and how or what he is doing.
4. Schedule outings for social activities and then follow through.

5. Do not convince yourself that you are the only one who can care for the patient.

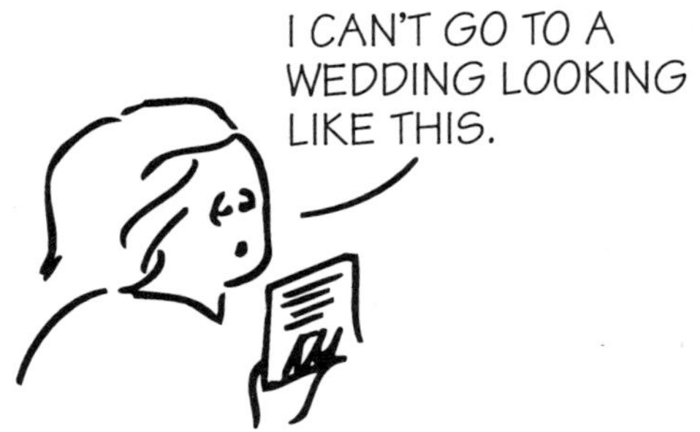

J. LEARNING TO LOVE AGAIN

Unless your loved one has only had a mild bump on the head (and sometimes even then), you will find that he is a somewhat different person from before. Now that he is being discharged you may be fantasizing that when he gets home he will be his "old self." You will be disappointed if you are expecting this, so please do not set yourself up for this letdown.

As time goes by you will probably note changes indicating that your loved one may never completely return to his original personality. You may feel that you are living or sleeping with a stranger. You will need time to adjust, so give yourself this opportunity. If it is your spouse who is injured, you may need to seek professional help to assist both of you in redeveloping your relationship.

EXAMPLES

1. The individual who is brain injured, who has always been the stronger of the two in the marriage relationship suddenly becomes dependent upon the other.

2. The older couple just beginning to enjoy retirement find themselves with the equivalent of a small child to care for, even though their son has been functioning independently for twenty years.

3. The woman who, prior to her husband's accident, played the dominant sexual role, finds that he is offended when she approaches him.
4. The mellow, mild-mannered husband has turned into a boisterous and offensive partner.
5. The previously active and exciting woman sits all day in front of a television and eats continuously.

RESOLUTIONS

1. Talk to him the way you used to.
2. Let him make as many decisions as possible.
3. Ask his opinion (even if it is not necessarily needed).
4. Approach the situation as you would a new relationship.

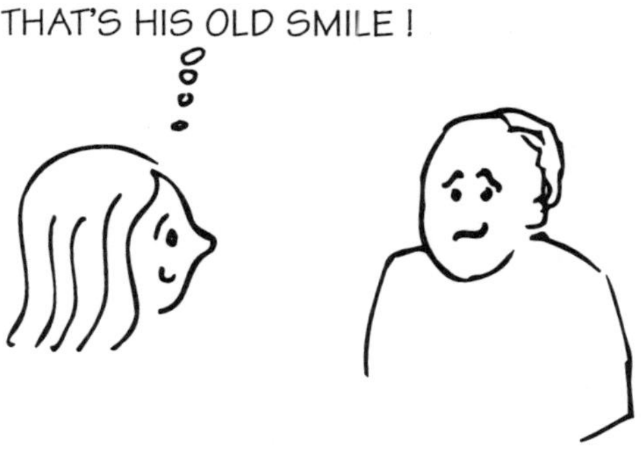

CONCLUSION

We hope that this manual has given you an idea of what to expect when you bring your loved one home, as well as provide some guidance for problem areas that may arise. If you are already caring for a loved one at home, we hope that the resolutions offered are of assistance in dealing with your family's specific problems. After reading this book we are sure you have realized that care in the home environment involves every family member and affects practically every aspect of family life. The family unit plays a critical role in the rehabilitation process, and understanding the reasons why certain behaviors and responses are triggered can help a great deal in adjusting to the pressures of bringing your loved one home.

Every family member will be changed by the accident - not just the person injured. It is important to recognize that things will never be the same as they were before the injury. But do not despair! Accepting this fact is the first step to creating and fostering a cohesive, loving family unit. Remember that life after brain injury can be productive and happy! Naturally, this is going to take work, patience and love from the whole family - whether that be the children, one spouse or a single parent. Good luck!